Intermittent Fasting

The Comprehensive and Sequential Manual for Achieving Weight Loss

(The Potential of Intermittent Fasting for Weight Reduction and Enhancing Health)

Mauricio Joseph

TABLE OF CONTENT

Stress-Induced Eating Habits... 1

No Dietary Restrictions, But A Fresh Start To Life! . 9

Smoothie With A Blend Of Avocado And Mango, Infused With Green Tea..34

Physical Hunger Vs. Psychological Hunger 35

Indulgent And Delectable Chocolate Chip Cheesecake Fat Treats 61

Advantages Of Intermittent Fasting............................63

Cauliflower Crust Pizza 86

Beverage Choices During Intermittent Fasting For Weight Loss 88

The Impact Of Intermittent Fasting On Weight Reduction 97

Lean Muscle Gain 101

STRESS-INDUCED EATING HABITS

Numerous individuals exhibit alterations in their dietary habits when exposed to heightened levels of stress. Let us expeditiously examine a few of these dietary modifications and their association with weight gain. Allow me to provide you with a concise overview:

The consumption of foods rich in fats and sugars is detrimental to health and often contributes to an increase in body weight. Primarily, these are processed food items characterized by their high sugar, sodium, and fat content. Regrettably, individuals have a tendency to desire these processed foods during periods of chronic stress, resulting in weight gain.

Engaging in emotional eating can be attributed to heightened levels of anxiety, excessive nervous energy, and an elevated cortisol production, which can result in an inclination towards consuming unhealthy food choices and an increased intake of food beyond one's typical consumption level. Upon indulging in a second serving or succumbing to emotional eating, you are likely to experience momentary alleviation of stress. In due course, one may notice an undesired increase in body fat and subsequent weight gain.

Consuming an increased amount of fast foods results in the abandonment of preparing a nutritionally balanced and wholesome dinner at home, leading to the consumption of fast foods that possess elevated levels of fat and sugar. Additionally, it is probable that under conditions of prolonged stress, you may engage in excessive consumption of food, particularly in larger quantities, without conscious awareness.

Experiencing a lack of time to engage in physical activity – it is important to acknowledge that a primary factor contributing to pervasive stress among individuals is the presence of overwhelming and demanding daily routines. This implies that physical activity is the least of their priorities, and it is completely absent from their agenda or list of tasks. Extensive work schedules, burdening commute, and engaging in sedentary activities upon returning home, severely restrict opportunities for engaging in physical exercise. Consequently, this results in an increase in body weight. Failure to consume an adequate amount of water leads to a perplexing correlation of thirst and hunger amidst a busy agenda, as one attempts to handle a myriad of life's obstacles. The ultimate outcome is an increase in caloric intake accompanied by insufficient hydration, consequently resulting in weight gain stemming from excessive overconsumption.

Omitting meals - you forgo consuming your breakfast in order to avoid being tardy for work or neglect consuming your lunch due to a multitude of tasks demanding your attention. The act of consuming a nutritious meal has ceased to remain a priority due to the challenges faced in managing a multitude of tasks within a hectic and demanding schedule. This level of stress can lead to excessive and unconscious overeating, as there is uncertainty regarding the availability of future eating opportunities.

Engaging in trendy diets - upon recognizing weight gain, individuals find themselves trapped in a recurring cycle of stress. You discover yourself engaging in injurious trendy dieting practices or restricting your food intake below your body's necessary level in an endeavor to reduce the surplus weight. You inadvertently overlooked the importance of consuming a well-rounded and nutritionally diverse meal containing carbohydrates, proteins, vegetables, and fruits. Whilst these perilous dietary regimens may initially captivate, they invariably pose a detriment to one's long-term well-being. These factors contribute to compulsive eating driven by emotions and lack of mindfulness, ultimately resulting in additional weight gain.

Sleep deprivation is commonly observed among individuals experiencing stress, leading to insomnia whereby one stays awake during the night, preoccupied with concerns such as overwhelming schedules, interpersonal dynamics, and parental responsibilities. Their strength of determination is diminished, and their metabolic rate decelerates as a result of sleep deprivation. The consequences of failing to practice mindful eating include the adoption of emotional eating behaviors, subsequently resulting in an increase in body weight.

Disrupting the cycle of stress and weight gain Alleviating the cycle of stress and weight gain Halting the cycle of stress and weight gain Interrupting the cycle of stress and weight gain Preventing the cycle of stress and weight gain

Breaking the cycle of stress and weight gain proves to be a formidable challenge. This occurs due to the recognition of weight gain and the resulting ill fit of clothing, thereby exacerbating the cycle of stress. It is important to bear in mind that heightened stress levels can render individuals more prone to weight gain. The ability to overcome this cycle will require determination. However, it is possible to mitigate the effects of stress along with the accompanying weight fluctuations by implementing certain actionable measures.

Place a strong emphasis on incorporating exercise into your daily routine – exercise plays a paramount role in alleviating stress and managing unwanted weight gain. Concurrently, physical activity has the ability to alleviate stress, while preventing any associated weight gain. Sustain a regular regimen of physical activity subsequent to the conclusion of your workday, whether through embarking on a jog in the vicinity, attending a fitness facility, or indulging in a leisurely stroll during the evening hours. Engaging in aerobic exercises proves to be the most efficacious approach in addressing weight gain caused by stress.

Pay attention to your dietary practices - being mindful of your food choices is crucial in order to manage and regulate your consumption patterns effectively. Cease engaging in emotional and mindless eating through the practice of maintaining a food journal. It would be beneficial for you to maintain a record of your dietary intake, either in the form of a food diary or through the utilization of a dedicated application to track your eating patterns. By conscientiously considering each food item consumed, you will have the opportunity to enhance your dietary choices and make improvements to your eating habits. Establish a dietary regimen and diligently organize nutritious meals for oneself in the comfort of one's own residence.

Engage in alternative fulfilling pursuits that are unrelated to sustenance – the presence of alternative activities can serve as a means to alleviate stress, reducing the likelihood of excessive food consumption. No matter how demanding your schedule may be, it is imperative that you allocate a portion of your time for relaxation and stress alleviation. Doing so will enable you to enhance your emotional state, rejuvenate your cognitive abilities, and enhance your mental clarity. One may choose to engage in activities such as receiving a massage, allocating time for socializing with friends and family, offering affection to one's canine companion, immersing oneself in literature, embarking on a hiking excursion, or participating in a yoga session. Participating in such activities can aid in the prevention of weight gain associated with stress and break the cycle of stress triggered by demanding schedules or any other sources of stress in your life.

No Dietary Restrictions, But A Fresh Start To Life!

Intermittent fasting moderately alters one's lifestyle. One acquires the ability to decline requests within designated time frames, and one's acquaintances demonstrate understanding and encouragement upon recognizing one's unequivocal commitment.

It is crucial to ensure that you obtain adequate rest throughout the fasting hours. Many individuals fail to recognize the true impact of adequate sleep. While in the state of slumber, metabolic processes result in the consumption of calories, while concurrently facilitating restorative function within the body. Therefore, given that you are providing your body with reduced nourishment, it is crucial to approach your sleep hours with utmost importance. Ensure that you obtain a minimum of eight hours of restful sleep as it aids in facilitating the fasting period and promotes rejuvenation upon awakening.

Engaging in a moderate level of physical activity can have positive effects on your well-being during a fasting period. Given the aim of achieving weight loss and improved physical fitness, engaging in rigorous physical activity before the evening meal or, if suitable, before lunch may be the most opportune time, considering personal preferences and schedule. If exercise doesn't appeal to you greatly, there are numerous enjoyable physical activities available that can be perceived as recreational rather than burdensome tasks. As an illustration, the possession of a Zumba-style dance DVD serves as a remarkable motivator to rise from a seated position and engage in a physical activity that promotes comprehensive bodily exercise. It provides enjoyment, thereby masking its nature as physical activity. In a similar vein, engaging in the act of regularly walking the dog serves as a beneficial means of attaining exercise that positively impacts cardiovascular well-being. Engaging in walking is consistently beneficial as it facilitates the activation of various body parts in a highly advantageous manner for one's overall health.

You might be curious about suitable beverage options during periods of fasting, and after careful consideration, I have discovered that nettle tea proves to be the most optimal choice. It possesses a sweetness that obviates the need for the inclusion of milk. Nonetheless, it is permissible to consume infusions or teas without the addition of milk or sugar, and it is advisable to experiment with various options until discovering a preferred choice.

If one tends to undervalue the efficacy of water consumption, it is pertinent to alter one's perspective. A substantial portion of the discomfort experienced by individuals who are overweight can be mitigated through the regular consumption of water, and this also holds true during mornings when limited alternatives are available for breakfast. Water aids in the process of purging the system, in addition to serving another function. It provides nourishment to your muscles and prevents their contraction due to dehydration. When instructing on the concept of intermittent fasting, I consistently encounter individuals who tend to disregard dehydration as a possible source of their discomfort, which never fails to astound me. They perceive this as an exceptionally significant event that is exclusive to individuals receiving medical care in hospitals. Regrettably, the inadequate consumption of water has a substantial impact on your internal state, regardless of your acknowledgment of it. Your body requires adequate hydration consistently.

An activity that I also highly advocate individuals to experiment with during their period of fasting is the practice of meditation. This aids in their relaxation and enhances their overall cognizance of the bodily transformations occurring. Fasting ceases to pose as a challenge. It is perceived as a form of philanthropy, and individuals who engage in meditation can effectively maintain composure and concentration towards their consistently beneficial dietary practices. They are also less predisposed to engage in dishonest behavior. The tranquility obtained through meditation significantly facilitates the entire process, particularly if one chooses to refrain from consuming food for a duration of 24 hours. The sustenance typically derived from food can be acquired through meditation, which holds significant value when enduring an extended fasting period.

It is imperative that you make adequate preparations for your dietary regimen and possess the necessary psychological resilience to effectively traverse the fasting duration, thereby mitigating any excessive unease or preoccupation with the need for sustenance. During the initial few days, you might experience fleeting sensations of hunger. However, because you are aware that sustenance will be available to you shortly, this is generally a manageable condition to overcome. If you are experiencing difficulty in managing the final hours of a fast, incorporating meditation into your practice could be beneficial.

What Anticipate When Commencing your Fresh Expedition of Existence

Establishing clear expectations prior to embarking on a period of fasting is a commendable approach to properly aligning your physical and mental preparedness for the forthcoming adjustments in lifestyle and dietary habits.

Prior to delving into the intricate nuances of these expectations, it is crucial to establish clarity regarding your personal objectives for the duration of the fast. The following are typical instances in which individuals have chosen to engage in fasting:

They aspire to shed pounds and attain a more slender physique.

They have previously experimented with alternative well-known dietary plans, expressing discontentment towards the procedure or vexation regarding the outcomes.

They have a strong desire to substantially enhance the present state of their physique.

Their desire is to experience an extended duration of existence, characterized by enhanced physical well-being and increased levels of productivity.

Fasting has been empirically demonstrated as an effective strategy for attaining weight loss in a manner conducive to overall well-being, simultaneously leading to heightened levels of energy. For numerous individuals, this practice holds profound transformative power, facilitating the attainment of their myriad personal ambitions.

Embracing a period of fasting necessitates unwavering resolve and self-assurance that you will persist steadfastly, resisting any temptation to revert to prior habits. It is imperative to develop a comprehensive strategy to effectively prepare for the situation at hand, as it may necessitate significant alterations to various aspects of your life.

For the purpose of your informed understanding, a comprehensive outline shall be presented delineating the assorted aspects that one ought to anticipate upon embarking on a fast:

Grocery Shopping

Fasting would bring about a substantial alteration in your approach to food shopping. In addition to addressing the frequency of your shopping days, it is necessary to remove certain items from your current shopping list and substitute them with healthier alternatives.

As a general rule, it is advisable to adhere to protein sources that are lower in fat content, primarily including select varieties of fish and egg whites. For fruits and vegetables, it is recommended to allocate a slightly higher budget and opt for organically grown produce.

Meal Restrictions

The specific meal schedule that one must adhere to is contingent upon the fasting method being undertaken. Nevertheless, each fasting technique entails restricting your calorie consumption, whether through the reduction of permissible caloric intake or the encouragement to forgo certain meals, if not all.

As an illustration, one can consider the 5:2 diet which entails a prescribed intake restriction of 500 calories for women, and 600 calories for men. Both quantities fall well below the recommended intake for the average person.

Consumption of alcoholic beverages while observing a period of fasting is strongly advised against. Even during periods of respite from fasting, professionals advise consuming only a moderate quantity.

Concurrently with the fasting period, it is imperative to increase your water intake. If your inclination leans towards flavored beverages, it would be advisable to opt for herbal teas and unsweetened black coffee. In addition, certain health professionals permit the consumption of club soda while observing a fast.

For further insight into the dietary constraints associated with various fasting methodologies, please consult chapter 4 of this publication.

Physiological side-effects

A number of these aforementioned side effects can be regarded as the drawbacks or unfavorable aspects of fasting. Nevertheless, by adopting the appropriate mindset, one can persevere through these obstacles, irrespective of the difficulties they may present in one's daily existence.

Hunger Pangs

Hunger is an inherent physiological response that arises when one initiates a period of refraining from food. It constitutes an inherent part of the fasting experience, albeit possessing elements that are not entirely adverse.

Research indicates that hunger has the potential to heighten cognitive concentration and enhance mental acuity, as supported by empirical findings.

Lightheadedness

It could potentially require a period of adjustment for you to become accustomed to being in a state of fasting. Throughout the transitional phase, it is probable that you will encounter sensations of lightheadedness and various other physical discomforts. Those symptoms are entirely within the range of what is considered normal, and they will dissipate as soon as your body has fully acclimated to the modifications in your routine.

Low Energy

Experiencing a decline in your energy levels is another transient symptom that you should anticipate and make arrangements for during the initial phases of your fasting period.

Your physique is accustomed to receiving a specific caloric intake on a daily basis. When the practice of omitting meals is initiated, the body would necessitate adaptation and engage various internal mechanisms in order to generate the necessary energy for normal functioning.

As per the analysis of professionals, this phase characterized by diminished energy levels may persist for a duration spanning one to two weeks. Subsequently, you would experience heightened vitality despite the continuation of fasting.

It is crucial to acquire the knowledge and skills necessary to adequately equip oneself for this advantageous transformation in one's life. It is advisable to adopt a low-carbohydrate, high-fat diet for a period of three weeks in order to commence intermittent fasting. It enables the body to utilize lipids instead of carbohydrates as a source of energy. This entails the exclusion of all sugars, cereals (such as bread, cookies, pasta, and rice), vegetables, and refined oils from the regimen. This will help to mitigate the most acute side effects.

Commence with a briefer duration of 16 hours, for example, commencing at the evening meal (8 pm) and concluding at midday the following day (12 pm). Typically, you will partake in meals during the hours of 12 pm to 8 pm, consuming two to three servings. Once you have become accustomed to it, you have the ability to expeditiously increase the duration to 18 or even 20 hours.

For briefer durations of fasting, you may engage in this practice consistently on a daily basis. For more protracted fasts ranging from 24-36 hours, it is recommended to engage in this practice on a weekly basis, allocating 1-3 days for fasting while alternating with regular eating days.

In order to provide a more comprehensive understanding of the experience one would undergo during a fasting regime, it is beneficial to present a detailed outline of a typical intermittent and extended fasting duration.

Your body will transition into a fasting state approximately eight hours following your most recent meal. This timeframe represents the typical duration required for the complete breakdown and assimilation of nutrients derived from the ingestion of food and beverages preceding your period of fasting.

The duration may differ, nonetheless, contingent upon the type of meal consumed; for instance, meals rich in fiber necessitate an extended period for digestion when contrasted with leafy vegetables.

Throughout the initial fasting phase, the primary source of energy for your body would continue to be derived from your glucose or glycogen reserves.

After an overnight fast, the glycogen reserves in your liver would become exhausted.

After the depletion of all the glucose reserves in your body, it would initiate the utilization of energy from the adipose tissue located within your body.

Please be aware that the body initiates the process of converting fat into energy prior to the complete depletion of glycogen stores within the body. Fasting concomitantly augments the process of lipolysis, thereby serving as an efficacious method for reducing surplus body mass.

There is no correct fasting regimen. The pivotal factor is to select the one that is most effective for your needs. Certain individuals may achieve favorable outcomes from briefer periods of fasting, while for others, longer durations of fasting may be necessary. Certain individuals opt for the traditional method of water purification, while others prefer expediting the process by making tea, coffee, or preparing bone broth. Irrespective of your actions, it is paramount to maintain proper hydration and diligently observe your well-being. It is advisable to cease any activity promptly if you experience any symptoms of illness. You may experience hunger, but do not suffer from any feelings of nausea.

Having an understanding of the anticipated outcomes is of utmost importance in ensuring the enduring success of your rapid progress. In view of the insights garnered from this chapter, reshape your objectives to develop a fasting regimen that is both pragmatic and attainable.

Hormonal factors and managing your overall well-being

The female gender entails multiple fundamental yet crucial responsibilities interconnected with caloric intake and the metabolic processes of the body. At its most fundamental essence, the female physique has been refined and honed throughout history to serve the purpose of fertility and human procreation. The process of abstaining from food, commonly known as fasting, has been observed to have a distinct impact on hormonal fluctuations in the female body, particularly among those who have not previously experienced fasting. These hormonal alterations differ from those observed in the male body. Presented below is a more in-depth analysis of the hormones that are influenced by Intermittent Fasting, along with strategies for women to recognize and counteract any alterations.

Estrogen & Progesterone

An imbalance in estrogen levels poses a significant health issue for females across all age groups. Estrogen and progesterone are essential hormones for maintaining overall physical well-being in females, making it crucial to ensure that these hormones are balanced within the body. Estrogen and progesterone play integral roles in various physiological processes in women, including metabolic regulation, cognitive functioning, stress and anxiety management, and overall emotional equilibrium.

Potential indicators of imbalanced estrogen levels include:

Decreased levels of energy and heightened muscular fatigue.

Reduced overall bone density and muscle firmness Diminished overall bone density and muscle tone Lowered total bone density and muscle tonicity Diminished total bone density and muscle muscularity

Reproductive disorders such as infertility and disturbances in menstrual patterns

Heightened body mass and elevated glucose levels

In the case of women attempting to conceive, an imbalance in estrogen due to decreased caloric intake can potentially impact the menstrual cycle and lead to progressive reduction in ovarian size. Despite the limited number of tests specifically examining the effects of fasting on women's health, in-depth research has been conducted on female rodents to investigate the physiological responses of their bodies during fasting intervals, particularly concerning hormonal equilibrium and reproductive abilities. These studies indicated that, within a period of two weeks following the commencement of fasting, certain female participants experienced decreased estrogen levels, diminished fertility, and reduced ovarian size, while others demonstrated minimal or negligible alterations.

This phenomenon occurs due to extended or variable durations of fasting, which can trigger a survival response mechanism in the female body. This innate desire to prioritize survival prompts the physique to refrain from expending valuable energy on non-essential tasks such as preparing for an unexpected pregnancy, and instead channel it more efficiently towards sustaining essential bodily functions. Hence, it is imperative for women who are contemplating pregnancy within the foreseeable future to adhere to a balanced diet and maintain an appropriate calorie intake, aligned with their specific body type and weight.

An additional factor that women ought to consider when assessing the impact of fasting on their hormone levels is the possibility of one hormonal imbalance triggering another. In the majority of instances where females have presented concerns regarding their estrogen levels, it has been observed that such imbalances have either initiated or exacerbated an underlying hormonal imbalance within the thyroid gland. The thyroid gland, located in the neck, is of utmost importance as it is intricately linked to the physiological mechanism of the body's metabolic activities. Thyroid hormone imbalances can exert adverse effects on metabolic processes and their functionality.

Regarding hormonal health and balance in relation to Intermittent Fasting for women, it is a complex subject whereby the body's response to fasting cannot be predetermined. To ascertain the genuine effects of Intermittent Fasting on your body, it is imperative to devise a meticulously informed plan and diligently adhere to your selected schedule for a duration of two weeks. Only then will you be able to discern any potential alterations or observations.

Smoothie With A Blend Of Avocado And Mango, Infused With Green Tea

Ingredients:

- 2 cups spinach, torn
- A pinch of sea salt
- **Stevia to taste (optional)**
- 2 cups green tea
- 1 medium avocado, peeled, pitted, cubed
- 1 tbsp coconut oil
- 2 cups mango chunks

Method:
1. Add all the ingredients in a blender and blend until smooth.
2. Pour into glasses and serve.

Physical Hunger Vs. Psychological Hunger

The primary deterrent to fasting for individuals is the concept of experiencing hunger. There exists a prevailing belief among individuals that if they refrain from consuming food, they will experience sensations of hunger and physical debilitation. It has transitioned into a psychological concern as opposed to a purely physical condition.

The prevailing scientific consensus suggests that individuals should consume four to six modest meals on a daily basis. For a considerable duration, adhering to a customary practice of consuming three standardized meals, namely breakfast, lunch, and dinner, has been the norm. During the intervals between those main meals, it is customary to consume one or two light snacks. It has become customary that individuals who have not eaten for a period of four to six hours are generally assumed to be experiencing hunger.

Hunger is an experience characterized by the occurrence of stomach growling and hunger pangs. Physical hunger arises as a result of various factors including the actions of the hypothalamus, the levels of blood glucose, the contents within the stomach and intestines, as well as the presence of specific hormones within the body. Prolonged deprivation of food could potentially result in symptoms such as headache, vertigo, and impaired cognitive focus.

A multitude of individuals experience anxiety when they begin to feel hunger. However, hunger is merely a sensation. Consider the early humans of prehistoric times, who did not adhere to structured meal times. They solely consumed sustenance when it was obtainable, given their need to engage in the pursuit of acquiring nourishment. However, they persevered due to the utilization of their stored fat reserves within their bodies.

Conversely, psychological hunger, referred to as "emotional hunger" as well, entails the act of consuming food not due to physical hunger, but to gratify specific emotional needs. It is associated with a desire. It arises abruptly and manifests as a strong desire for certain types of foods.

For the purpose of enhanced comprehension, a juxtaposition of the ensuing developments during physiological hunger and psychological hunger is presented below.

Consumption driven by physiological need.

PSYCHOLOGICAL HUNGER

It develops incrementally and can be postponed. It emerges abruptly and is characterized by its high intensity.

Any form of sustenance, whether nutritious or manufactured, will suffice and induce a sensation of satiety. Specific foods (eg. Baked goods and savory pies, such as cookies and pizza, evoke intense desires and fulfill emotional gratification.

Stops eating when full. Ceases consumption once the sensation or desire has dissipated or been dulled.

Feels nourished & content. Eliminates hunger pangs. Frequently culminates in sensations of culpability and remorse.

In the event that physiological hunger is inherently determined by biological factors and correlated with blood glucose levels, what stimuli elicit psychological eating?

Psychological hunger is instigated by a multitude of factors, including:

• Social interaction - the leading factor behind undesirable culinary behaviors. Social events and social gatherings often result in excessive consumption of food due to its availability. Individuals often resort to eating as a means to alleviate their nervousness, or as a way to engage with others in the group.

• Stress - the release of cortisol, a hormone associated with stress, induces a desire for confections, savory items, and foods high in fat content, thereby providing a temporary surge of energy and enjoyment during times of pressure.

• Emotional states – individuals may resort to food as a means of finding solace, indulging in self-reward, or commemorating joyous occasions, such as sadness, happiness, or excitement.

• Childhood customs – culinary delights that evoke nostalgic sentiment and are frequently linked to pleasant reminiscences (e.g. indulging in a sundae at the local ice cream emporium; enjoying a barbecue gathering with companions)

Strategies for Addressing Psychological Hunger

On subsequent occasions when experiencing a strong desire for indulgent fare, exercise patience for a duration of 10 minutes before succumbing to the temptation to partake in your favored comfort food. In most instances, the urge will diminish. Explore alternative options, such as engaging in a variety of activities or experimenting with a different sport. Leading a more health-conscious lifestyle facilitates the cultivation of nutritious and mindful eating habits, thereby fostering a sense of discipline when it comes to making wholesome dietary choices.

Through the practice of fasting, individuals can develop a heightened discernment between physiological hunger and psychological cravings. Upon the conclusion of the day or the designated period of fasting, reflect upon the sensation you are currently undergoing - which corresponds to genuine physical hunger within the body.

Additionally, you may consider acquainting yourself with the ensuing stages of hunger:

Level 1 – Starving. Dizzy. Disoriented.

Level 2 – Experiencing a significant degree of hunger. Extreme stomach grumbling. Cranky.

Level 3 – Hungry. Stomach growls a little.

Level 4 – Beginning to experience mild hunger pangs.

Level 5 – Satisfied. I am satiated, but do not possess a voracious appetite.

Chapter 3: Explore the Intriguing Scientific Principles of Fasting

Good-to-Know Medical Terminology:

Insulin responsiveness" "Insulin sensitivity status" "Degree of insulin sensitivity

In order to maintain the stability of your body's blood sugar levels, the functioning of insulin is relied upon by your body. When your level of sensitivity is diminished, it indicates that you possess a certain degree of resistance. Effective management of resistance necessitates an elevated amount of insulin in order to maintain adequate levels of blood sugar. The process of fasting can have an effect on insulin levels and blood sugar levels due to the fundamental influence of dietary choices on insulin production.

"Glucose"

Energy is generated upon the disintegration of this basic sugar compound. It is an essential carbohydrate for physiological functioning, though its regulation can be challenging. When individuals experience difficulties in maintaining proper regulation of their glucose levels, an excess amount of sugar accumulates within their bloodstream, surpassing the capacity of their bodies to manage effectively.

An instance of inflammatory response" or "The occurrence of inflammatory process

An infection or injury elicits a physiological reaction whereby the affected area exhibits erythema due to increased blood flow, accompanied by swelling resulting from the extravasation of cellular fluid to provide localized cushioning. Additionally, one would experience the sensation of increased warmth resulting from the augmented presence of the additional red blood cells swiftly flowing towards the affected area. During the period of fasting, one can observe a beneficial impact on the chronic inflammation present in the body, which serves no essential function for its defense.

"Biomarkers"

This is a diagnostic tool employed for the assessment of individuals' health conditions, specifically in identifying the presence of infections or diseases. Furthermore, this phrase is employed in discussions regarding the quantification of diseases affecting animals. In the context of fasting, this terminology is commonly employed to analyze the quantifiable factors preceding and subsequent to a fasting interval.

"Heterogeneous"

This implies the presence of variety in both the character and content. It is commonly employed to denote discrepancies in the outcomes of fasting experiences between individuals of the female and male genders.

"Metabolic"

The energy derived from the consumption of food is a combination of chemical and physiological processes within the human body. This system is of immense complexity, yet it plays a crucial role in fostering your well-being and ensuring your long life. Your metabolic rate is influenced by both your dietary and exercise practices.

"Angiogenesis"

This entails the generation of fresh blood cells within your organism. When one nourishes the body with appropriate nutrients, an increased production of blood cells ensues as opposed to periods of inadequate nutrition; however, the continual formation of blood vessels is an ongoing process in the human body. As you generate fresh vascular networks, you are directing their growth towards both the healthy regions of your body and those areas that are less optimal. As an illustration, in the case of a tumor or malignant growth, there is a process of vascularization in which new blood vessels are being nurtured to sustain and promote its growth. During the period of fasting, there is a curtailment of neovascularization, resulting in the deprivation of vital nourishment to undesirable regions of the body.

The autonomous nervous system

The autonomic nervous system encompasses an assortment of functions and organs, such as respiration, cardiac pulsation, and gastrointestinal activity. You are unable to exert conscious control over your autonomic nervous system. This implies that in the event of a malfunction in any of these systems, one must not contemplate ways to repair it; rather, a distinct mode of communication must be employed. Fasting is among the methods through which you can accomplish that objective.

Pertaining to the human or animal biological rhythm that follows a 24-hour cycle.

You possess an inherent, biological timing mechanism that naturally conforms to a 24-hour cycle. The regulation of your eating, sleeping, and daily activities is governed by this innate "circadian clock" or inherent rhythm.

Scientific Evidence regarding Fasting

Cancer

Undoubtedly, one of the most extensively studied domains concerning fasting pertains to its association with cancer prevention and healing. Senior Investigator Mark Mattson, affiliated with the National Institute of Aging, has authored a publication in the renowned Canadian Medical Association Journal. In this study, it was observed that fasting, especially intermittent fasting, yielded noteworthy favorable effects on the biomarkers associated with diverse diseases, encompassing various types of cancers. In a research conducted by Mattson, it was observed that implementing a restriction in caloric intake among subjects resulted in a deceleration of cancer progression. Furthermore, it was hypothesized that this phenomenon likely extends to human physiology. If you are employing fasting as a strategy to aid in the prevention or treatment of cancer, Mattson recommends refraining from excessive consumption of unhealthy foods outside the fasting periods.

However, he counsels that, drawing from the findings of his experiments conducted on mice, it would be prudent to direct your attention towards consuming a moderate quantity of calories during those periods, thereby maintaining a reduced overall caloric intake.

A peer-reviewed publication in the esteemed Journal of Midlife Health authored by Dr. Nair reveals that breast cancer ranks as the prevailing form of cancer globally. Breast cancer ranks as the second most prevalent cause of mortality among females with cancer-related deaths. Although primarily found in women, it can also impact males. Nair's research findings revealed a conspicuous correlation between fasting and the deceleration of tumor growth, as well as the tumor's receptiveness to concurrent treatments like chemotherapy. The findings of this article unambiguously indicate that fasting has the capacity to decelerate and potentially halt the progression of various diseases, including cancer. Additionally, it renders cancerous cells more vulnerable, thereby heightening their responsiveness to cancer treatments administered by healthcare practitioners for the specific tumor. The inhibition of angiogenesis is responsible for the deceleration or cessation of disease progression. A malignant neoplasm necessitates the formation of novel blood vessels to obtain nourishment. However, when deprived of this supply, the tumor's growth is hindered and ultimately it may succumb entirely.

Dr. Nair collaborated with other medical practitioners, including Brandhorst, Bianchi, Raffaghello, and Safdie. They authored a paper that was subsequently published in the Journal of Science of

Translational Medicine. In the course of this study, they observed the evolution of cancerous tumors in rodents. This study corroborated the conclusions outlined in Nair's aforementioned article, demonstrating the significant inhibitory effect of fasting on tumor development. Moreover, it accentuated the complementary role of fasting in enhancing various cancer treatments. However, the primary focus of these studies has predominantly been on animal subjects. Further investigation involving human subjects is imperative for comprehending the correlation between fasting and cancer. It is highly recommended to consult with your medical professionals prior to initiating a fasting regimen as part of your cancer treatment, in order to assess the potential merits and feasibility of such an approach. As per a publication in the Journal of Fasting Health, fasting is considered to be the "solution to cancer"; however, it is advisable to assess its suitability in accordance with your distinctive requirements and circumstances.

Diabetes

There exist two primary classifications of diabetes: Type 1, which manifests in early stages of life and is not influenced by weight, and Type 2, which develops later and is characterized by the body's diminished ability to adequately respond to glucose through appropriate insulin levels. This secondary form of diabetes is frequently associated with excessive body weight, typically concentrated in the abdominal region. Engaging in fasting may pose risks for individuals with Type 1 diabetes as the body may not possess a definitive mechanism to cease the ketosis process. However, under the supervision of a medical practitioner, it can potentially be beneficial. For individuals diagnosed with Type 2 diabetes, significant improvements can be achieved by reducing total body weight and diminishing waist circumference. According to a research article published in the Diabetes, Metabolic Syndrome, and Obesity Journal, individuals who engaged in a four-week fasting regimen experienced notable reductions in their total body weight, waist circumference, and Body Mass Index (BMI). Upon the occurrence of this event, their physiological response to insulin was heightened, leading to an enhanced capacity for blood sugar regulation. This, consequently, aided in the natural regulation of their diabetes. Certain participants achieved such significant outcomes in managing their diabetes that they were able to discontinue the administration of insulin injections altogether.

Dr. Mark Mattson and Dr. Valter Longo have authored a scholarly article in the distinguished journal, Cell Metabolism, elucidating the potential of fasting in mitigating the onset and management of diabetes. The identical findings were reached by the two physicians in this article. Fasting has the potential to mitigate the onset of diabetes by promoting natural blood sugar stabilization. Additionally, it can serve as a therapeutic measure by restoring the body to a state of homeostasis and enhancing its responsiveness to insulin. However, similar to the aforementioned research on cancer mentioned in the preceding section, the majority of these experiments are conducted on animal subjects. Further clinical investigations involving human subjects are imperative in order to establish fasting as a conclusive and efficacious method for the prevention and restoration of diabetes. Mattson and Longo explicate within this specific scholarly article that your cellular structures exhibit resemblance to your muscular system. When subjected to controlled stress within a regulated setting, such as a fitness facility, individuals can enhance their capacity to withstand and adapt to increased stress levels and physical demands. When deliberate cellular strain is induced, the cells develop increased resilience to effectively manage the imposed stress. The augmented potency facilitates the cellular capacity to combat intrusive ailments such as diabetes and cancer.

Obesity

On occasions, obesity can give rise to diabetes, although this correlation is not absolute. Being afflicted with obesity in isolation poses significant health risks, while concurrently serving as a precipitant for various grave ailments that necessitate prudent attention. According to the study published in the Journal of American Board of Family Medicine, obesity has been found to be associated with several other conditions such as impaired fertility, osteoarthritis, chronic lower back pain, and coronary artery disease. Cancer is additionally more common in individuals who are obese. Numerous associations exist between various forms of cancer and obesity. Furthermore, it is worth noting that individuals affected by obesity also experience significant effects on their mental well-being. There exists a multitude of factors through which obesity can potentially exert an impact on an individual's mental well-being, but arguably the most salient link can be established with society's prevailing standards of an idealized body image. Due to the pervasive influence of media and messaging, individuals afflicted with obesity often experience diminished self-esteem and psychological distress, such as depression.

The efficacy of fasting as a means of achieving weight loss has been reported in numerous scholarly journals. As an illustration, Krista Varady, a distinguished researcher from the Department of Kinesiology and Nutrition at the University of Illinois at Chicago, delivered a comprehensive presentation on various strategies employed for weight reduction, notably fasting, and its proven efficacy. A further publication authored by Varady in Obesity Reviews has identified fasting as a viable method for weight reduction. Furthermore, the second article effectively exemplified the efficacy of fasting as a more superior approach for weight loss in comparison to various alternative methods. This phenomenon can be attributed to the preservation of lean mass, such as muscles and bone, coupled with the reduction of fat mass or fat storage.

Dr. Mark Mattson and Dr. Valter Longo elucidated in a separate publication in Cell Metabolism that fasting is a practicable approach that the majority of individuals can readily incorporate into their everyday routine. They elaborated on the notion that fasting constituted a commendable approach towards attaining optimal health, particularly for individuals grappling with overweight or obesity, citing its abundant advantages. By making alterations to both your lifestyle and dietary habits, you have the ability to mitigate nearly all of the potential hazards linked to obesity, while simultaneously decreasing your overall body mass. Numerous healthcare professionals and scholars have increasingly embraced the notion of fasting as a viable remedy for obesity. This is particularly due to its potential for long-term sustenance and consistently reproducible outcomes across diverse individuals and circumstances.

Indulgent And Delectable Chocolate Chip Cheesecake Fat Treats

Ingredient List:

- Chocolate chips- ex. Lily's sweetened with stevia (.25 cup)
- Vanilla extract (1 tsp.)
- Unchilled cream cheese - softened (4 oz.)
- Melted butter (4 tbsp.)
- Coconut oil (.25 cup)
- Sweetener ex. Lakanto Monkfruit (2 tbsp.)

Ensure the mini cupcake pan is appropriately prepared, either by with the use of liners or without them.

Incorporate the liquified butter, cream cheese, coconut oil, sweetener, and vanilla extract together in a mixing vessel.

Using a hand mixer, thoroughly combine the ingredients for a duration of two to three minutes until a smooth consistency is achieved.

Gently incorporate the chocolate chips into the mixture, reserving a few for optional garnishing on each bomb.

Transfer the mixture into the cavities of the muffin tin.

Freeze for 30 minutes. Please transfer from the tray and proceed with serving.

Advantages Of Intermittent Fasting

In addition to the aforementioned considerations regarding weight loss and heightened energy levels, intermittent fasting does entail other advantages, namely the ensuing:

1: It enhances the immune system and mitigates inflammation.

If you have conducted a thorough inquiry into intermittent fasting, you would have undoubtedly encountered assertions regarding its effectiveness in the reduction of inflammation, as well as its potent capabilities in significant enhancements of immunity and tissue recuperation.

The occurrence is that intermittent fasting acts as a catalyst in initiating the process of immune system regeneration, by stimulating the body to generate new white blood cells. When an individual engages in self-imposed starvation, it triggers a physiological response within the body where the system attempts to conserve energy. In this particular instance, one of the measures it takes to ensure this outcome is the recycling of numerous immune cells that are deemed unnecessary, specifically those that may be susceptible to damage (which is why there is a noticeable decrease in white blood cell count as observed in various studies exploring the effects of extended fasting). Upon resuming consumption of food, the blood cells are restored.

To clarify, it should be noted that the reduction of white blood cells prompts the regenerative process of producing new cells in the immune system through the use of stem cells. The gene PKA is responsible for inducing a state of regeneration in the stem cells, prompting them to enter a dormant phase. Consider it the signal for the stem cells to commence proliferation and undertake the task of regenerating the entire system. It may be of interest to note that PKA has also been linked to the process of aging, heightened tumor proliferation, and the development of cancer.

Furthermore, intermittent fasting effectively regulates the secretion of inflammatory cytokines within the body, including prominent ones like Tumor Necrosis Factor Alpha and Interleukin-6. Both of these agents contribute to an inflammatory response within the body, and fasting serves to diminish their release, thereby enhancing the robustness of the immune system.

If individuals are experiencing allergies and autoimmune disorders such as rheumatoid arthritis, systemic lupus,

Crohn's disease, and colitis, the immune system modulation associated with intermittent fasting (IF) can significantly contribute to managing these conditions. IF effectively alleviates the excessive inflammatory responses, thus promoting a more balanced immune function and enhancing overall condition management. When considering prevalent illnesses such as cancer, it is crucial to acknowledge that cancer cells possess a significantly higher number of insulin receptors compared to healthy cells. The estimated ratio ranges from ten to seventy times more insulin receptors on cancerous cells, resulting in their dependency on glucose as a source of energy. As you may be aware, the implementation of intermittent fasting demonstrates the capacity to diminish blood sugar levels, thereby depriving cancerous cells of necessary sustenance. Consequently, this weakened state renders them susceptible to impairment caused by free radicals and eventual annihilation.

2: Mitigate the effects of oxidative stress to counteract aging and various disease processes, while concurrently facilitating the regeneration and recuperation of bodily tissues.

The process of aging occurs as a result of cellular damage caused by oxidative stress. Therefore, implementing measures to prevent and repair such damage can be highly beneficial in counteracting the aging process.

Should you have any queries, the stress being alluded to in this context pertains to the situation wherein there is an elevated generation of free radicals beyond the usual levels, such as oxygen reactive species. These molecules, in essence, are inherently unstable and typically bear reactive electrons. The response observed bears resemblance to that of an oxidative process, akin to the phenomenon of rusting. In the present context, when your body cells come into contact with such reactions, they undergo a process akin to cellular corrosion.

How it happens

When encountering another molecule, one of these free radicals either relinquishes an electron or acquires one from it. This phenomenon has the potential to readily initiate a swift cascade whereby electrons are yielded or extracted among molecules, resulting in the formation of additional free radicals. The issue at hand is that these substances are capable of severing bonds between atoms within critical cellular constituents, including the cellular membrane, DNA, and vital proteins. The evident outcome entails accelerated aging and susceptibility to illness.

Allow me to provide you with a contextual understanding - oxidative stress has the potential to give rise to:

Cancer

Alzheimer's disease

Neurodegeneration

Diabetes

Cardiovascular disease

Cataracts

Arthritis

Autoimmune conditions

Fatigue

Brain fog

Wrinkles

Grey hair

Worsening eyesight

Depressed immunity

It is necessary to acknowledge that the malfunctioning of mitochondria, which are cellular organelles responsible for energy production, can lead to the generation of free radicals. When transitioning from a regular eating pattern to fasting, the cells experience restricted availability of glucose and subsequently commence seeking alternative sources of energy, such as fatty acids - as you are already aware. Consequently, the cells have the capacity to activate survival mechanisms, enabling the elimination of malfunctioning mitochondria and gradually replenishing them with viable counterparts. This process effectively diminishes the production of free radicals.

Fasting also elicits an initial rise in free radicals, prompting cellular upregulation of endogenous antioxidants to counteract future oxidative stress. Despite the commonly held belief that free radicals are inherently detrimental due to their capacity to harm cells, they may serve as crucial momentary triggers within your body, stimulating cellular adaptation to more substantial future challenges in a more effective manner.

Please be advised that numerous individuals choose to utilize external antioxidants to rectify this process by translocating the necessary electrons in order to stabilize the free radicals prior to inflicting further damage to the body. Personally, I find fasting to be a more feasible option due to its innate compatibility with our natural physiological functions.

The function of human growth hormone (HGH)

Intermittent fasting additionally enhances the production of the human growth hormone (HGH), thereby exerting a potent anti-aging effect by effectively decelerating the rate of cellular aging. Upon the release of HGH within the body, the activation of repair mechanisms is automatically prompted. HGH primarily induces physiological changes in the body's metabolism, promoting the conservation of protein and the utilization of fat for energy. Your body utilizes amino acids and proteins to facilitate the restoration of tissue collagen, thereby enhancing the efficiency and resilience of tendons, muscles, bones, and ligaments. With a sufficient presence of HGH circulating in your bloodstream, your skin's functionality is enhanced, the appearance of wrinkles is diminished, and the process of healing cuts and burns is expedited.

3: Fasting Enhances Cognitive Function: Enhances Memory Retention, Enhances Mental Acuity (Reduces Cognitive Impairment), and Promotes Neurological Development.

To begin with, your endocrine system (the collection of glands that produce hormones) assists in balance and production of vital hormones thus assisting your body to grow and develop. Nevertheless, it is your brain that initiates the initial communication to regulate these hormones. The hypothalamus, referred to as the central regulatory region of the brain, routinely monitors hormone levels multiple times within a given day. This region of the brain maintains ongoing communication with the pituitary gland, facilitating the secretion of hormones by the thyroid, adrenal, and parathyroid glands. The thyroid glands play a direct role in the regulation of your metabolic processes. Metabolism refers to the body's ability to metabolize food and obtain energy from it. This gland accomplishes this by synthesizing two varieties of hormones, namely T3 and T4, which effectively govern the functioning of the system. These hormones remain in a perpetual state of flux due to the continuous transmission of signals originating from the brain. The functioning of your thyroid operates within a feedback mechanism, wherein your brain ensures the maintenance of an efficient metabolism.

The issue arises when an excessive amount of food is consumed, particularly those high in sugar or starch. This leads to a rapid increase in blood sugar levels, or the consumption of processed foods which the brain may not perceive as immediate fuel. These factors can disrupt the feedback loop, resulting in diminished functioning of the thyroid and brain, manifesting as sluggishness. Consequently, this results in a deceleration of your metabolic rate, diminished cognitive abilities, and gradual weight increase over time. Intermittent fasting guarantees a reduction in food intake, enhances insulin sensitivity through the decrease in insulin levels in the bloodstream, consequently promoting metabolic activity.

Cognitive functions and cognitive acuity.

As previously stated, intermittent fasting (IF) elevates the concentration of human growth hormone (HGH) within the bloodstream. Consequently, this phenomenon contributes to neural processing and synaptic functioning, thereby enhancing memory retention and cognitive efficiency. Research conducted by Intermountain Medical Center reveals that a brief period of fasting lasting 24 hours can significantly enhance the circulation of Human Growth Hormone (HGH), with a staggering increase of approximately 1,300 percent observed. For men specifically, this increase is even more remarkable, reaching around 2,000 percent.

When discussing cognitive impairment commonly known as brain fog, it has been determined that excessive sugar intake, typically resulting from overconsumption of food, is the primary contributing factor. The majority of individuals experience an abrupt surge followed by a subsequent state of exhaustion. The primary advantage of intermittent fasting in this regard lies in its ability to assist the brain in reducing its dependence on glucose as an energy source and instead shift towards a more sustainable energy supply derived from fats.

The neurological response to intermittent fasting has been compared to that evoked by physical exercise. These two activities have a significant impact on the augmentation of protein synthesis in the brain, thereby facilitating the enhancement of neuronal connectivity and growth, alongside fortifying synaptic resilience. Synapses serve as the intermediary connections between neurons, enabling effective communication and facilitating the orderly operation of the nervous system. More specifically, intermittent fasting promotes neurogenesis in the hippocampus, facilitates ketogenesis, and enhances mitochondrial biogenesis in neurons, thereby facilitating the preservation of neuronal connectivity. This collective outcome serves to enhance both memory retention and learning aptitude.

We could extensively discuss the advantageous effects of intermittent fasting on cognitive function and its potential to facilitate overall well-being. However, given the knowledge we have accumulated thus far, I believe you grasp the concept.

4: Enhances Women's Reproductive Well-being and Cardiac Function (Cardiovascular Health)

In recent years, there has been a widespread recognition of the effectiveness of fasting in enhancing reproductive health, making it a prevalent component of reproductive health treatment. To begin with, the adoption of intermittent fasting can lead to improvement or prevention of specific health conditions associated with endocrine dysfunction that have adverse effects on reproductive health, such as obesity, Polycystic Ovarian Syndrome (PCOS), and metabolic syndrome.

The majority of research carried out on this topic has established a correlation between Polycystic Ovary Syndrome (PCOS) and decreased levels of stress neurohormone (a hormone produced by specialized nervous tissues rather than the endocrine glands). This finding has been linked to potential benefits for both the physical and mental well-being of women affected by PCOS. Additionally, they undergo an elevation in the luteinizing hormone, which plays a crucial role in maintaining regular and healthy ovulation patterns. This indicates positive prospects in terms of hormone regulation and serves as an indicator of reproductive capability.

It is important to take into consideration that pregnant women are generally advised against engaging in any fasting practice. However, this does not imply that you are prohibited from doing so. If you happen to be expecting a child, you may make adjustments to your dietary choices during the designated feeding periods. As an illustration, it is advisable to augment your consumption of nourishing fats while concurrently limiting or moderating your intake of processed and refined grains throughout the duration of your pregnancy. It is advisable to seek guidance from your healthcare provider in order to determine the most suitable approach to intermittent fasting (refer to the subsequent section), to ensure the utmost well-being of your pregnancy.

Please be advised that a consensus among reputable experts in the field of dietetics, particularly those with a focus on pregnancy and fertility, currently exists in favor of prescribing a meticulously crafted dietary plan for pregnant individuals affected by gestational diabetes. This recommended regimen comprises a restricted carbohydrate intake coupled with an increased consumption of dietary fat. By utilizing these companion models of 'fasting,' you can ascertain their therapeutic benefits and safety without requiring expertise in rocket science.

What is the status of your cardiovascular well-being?

Familiar to you is cholesterol, a lipophilic compound that is synthesized by the liver in response to bodily needs and can also be obtained through dietary sources. Cholesterol is transported within the bloodstream via Low density lipoproteins (LDL) and High density lipoproteins (HDL). LDL, or low-density lipoprotein, is colloquially referred to as the bad cholesterol. Its function involves transporting cholesterol to fulfill the needs of various body regions. However, an excess amount of LDL in the bloodstream may lead to its accumulation within the walls of blood vessels, potentially resulting in their obstruction. This situation entails a potential hazard as the presence of narrowed or obstructed arteries poses a hindrance to the optimal circulation of blood towards vital organs such as the heart and brain. The outcome entails the occurrence of a heart attack, stroke, or potential onset of heart failure. Numerous studies, including this one that lasted eight weeks, have provided conclusive evidence of the significant correlation between elevated LDL levels and the risk of developing heart disease.

In contrast, the HDL is commonly referred to as the favorable cholesterol due to its absence of adverse effects exerted by the LDL, and its role in efficiently gathering cholesterol before facilitating its transportation to the liver for elimination. In order to maintain a state of good health, it is typically necessary to maintain elevated levels of HDL while concurrently keeping LDL levels low, thereby helping to lower the likelihood of developing heart disease.

Other studies have also demonstrated the significant impact that intermittent fasting can have in lowering LDL levels. During the duration of this 8-week study, we observed notable alterations in the physique of overweight and obese women who engaged in intermittent fasting, adhering to a regime of consuming only one meal (comprising 500 to 600 kcal) on the designated fast days. These individuals experienced substantial reductions in body fat and waist circumference, as well as improvements in blood pressure, blood glucose levels, and a notable decrease in low density lipoprotein (LDL) levels. Additional research has observed similar enhancements in cardiovascular risk indicators irrespective of individuals' adherence to a low-fat diet or a standard American diet during the designated eating periods. Further readings are available, both found here and here.

We possess numerous additional advantages associated with intermittent fasting that fall outside the purview of this book. In essence, intermittent fasting offers the most optimal means by which to attain improved health and well-being in a natural manner.

Now, let us proceed to examine how you can implement this dietary regimen.

Cauliflower Crust Pizza

- 2 medium eggs
- 1 Tsp salt
- 2 cups mozzarella cheese grated
- 1 medium cauliflower head
- ½ cup grated parmesan cheese
- Italian seasoning

Method

Using a food processor, carefully blend the cauliflower florets until they achieve a powdered consistency. Please transfer the powder into a bowl, ensure it is covered, and proceed to heat it in the microwave until it achieves a soft consistency, which should take approximately 4 or 5 minutes. Transfer the mixture onto a pristine kitchen towel and permit it to cool.

Once the mixture has cooled to a manageable temperature, hold onto the kitchen towel and apply pressure to extract as much moisture as possible. Incorporate the remaining ingredients into a sizable bowl. Obtain a baking sheet and place a layer of parchment paper on top. Transfer the mixture onto the baking sheet and exert pressure to mold it into a circular form.

Place in an oven that has been pre-heated to a temperature of 400 degrees Fahrenheit and bake for a duration of 15 minutes, or until the desired golden color is achieved. Remove the pizza base from the oven and you'll have a guilt-free final product. Garnish with your preferred sauce and incorporate your favored toppings. Complement your dining experience with a nutritious salad to create a satisfying repast.

Beverage Choices During Intermittent Fasting For Weight Loss

1. Tea

If you possess an affinity for tea, you will find solace in the fact that this warm beverage seamlessly aligns with the objectives of intermittent fasting. Following are the advantages associated with this:

It facilitates the reduction of hunger" "It aids in diminishing hunger" "It contributes to the alleviation of hunger" "It supports the mitigation of hunger

This is a crucial aspect. When our food consumption is reduced, we experience sensations of hunger. This phenomenon can be attributed to an imbalance in the hunger hormone, ghrelin. We must return to this equilibrium if we desire to experience diminished hunger.

One possible alternative in a formal tone could be: "The catechins found in green tea, along with other compounds, serve the purpose of modulating the concentration of ghrelin within the human body."

Alternatively, with the passage of time, the level of ghrelin will diminish organically. The more restraints imposed on one's food intake, the fewer levels of ghrelin are synthesized.

It facilitates the process of weight reduction.

Various types of tea have the potential to exert a positive impact on weight reduction.

a) The presence of catechins in green tea induces the combustion of visceral adipose tissue, specifically the adipose tissue located in the abdominal region. Accumulating this kind of fat can elevate the susceptibility to insulin resistance and type 2 diabetes.

b) Additional research has indicated that white tea demonstrates comparable efficacy to green tea in terms of reducing visceral fat.

c) The synergy between catechins and caffeine present in green and white teas serves to enhance metabolic activity, resulting in potential increments of up to 4% in certain instances. Maintaining an efficient metabolic rate facilitates enhanced calorie expenditure throughout the day.

2.Coffee

This product comprises caffeine, renowned for its stimulating effects on awareness and its ability to suppress appetite. Furthermore, caffeine enhances metabolism and facilitates weight reduction.

Hence, consuming coffee is a commendable approach to manage appetite and enhance fat oxidation during the fasting period.

3. Apple cider vinegar (ACV),

Apple cider vinegar primarily consists of water and acid compounds, specifically acetic acid and malic acid. A volume of 15 ml (equivalent to one tablespoon) of apple cider vinegar is estimated to contain approximately 3 calories. Perfect for weightloss!

OPTIONS FOR BEVERAGES: IMPLEMENTING INTERMITTENT FASTING TO INDUCE AUTOPHAGY.

Autophagy is a physiological mechanism of the human body involving the degradation and elimination of aged or impaired cells. If these cells persist within the body, they elicit inflammation, subsequently resulting in various health complications.

The practice of intermittent fasting serves to stimulate the process of autophagy, which aids in the purification of the organism.

Green tea contains active polyphenols like epigallocatechin gallate (EGCG) in addition to caffeine, which collectively provide an additional stimulation to autophagy.

Bone broth, when incorporated into an intermittent fasting regimen, yields benefits such as improved skin complexion, enhanced hair and nail health, diminished inflammation, and a decelerated aging process.

Regardless of whether your objective is weight loss or overall health improvement, the inclusion of bone broth in your dietary regimen is absolutely essential.

Which individuals are advised against engaging in intermittent fasting?

Women seeking to conceive, currently experiencing pregnancy, or engaged in breastfeeding.

Individuals who are suffering from malnutrition or experiencing inadequate body weight.

Minors below the age of 18 and individuals who are advanced in age.

Those who have gout.

Individuals afflicted with gastroesophageal reflux disease (GERD).

Individuals who are afflicted with eating disorders should initially seek consultation with their physicians.

Individuals who are currently on diabetic medications and insulin should seek prior consultation with their healthcare providers, as adjustments in dosage may be necessary.

Individuals who are currently undergoing medication should seek advice from their physicians before making any changes as it may potentially impact the timing of their medication.

Individuals experiencing high levels of stress or issues related to cortisol should refrain from fasting, as it can serve as an additional stressor.

Individuals who engage in rigorous training on a daily basis should refrain from fasting.

If pertaining to women aged 50 years or older?

It is evident that our bodies and metabolism undergo transformations upon entering menopause. One notable transformation observed among women aged 50 and older is a decrease in metabolic rate, leading to weight gain. Engaging in fasting can potentially serve as an effective method for reversing and preemptively avoiding this weight gain. Research has indicated that the adoption of this fasting regimen contributes to the management of one's appetite, resulting in reduced cravings compared to individuals who do not abide by this practice consistently. If you are beyond the age of 50 and seeking to adapt to your decelerated metabolic rate, intermittent fasting can assist in preventing excessive daily food consumption.

At the age of 50, individuals may begin to experience the onset of certain chronic conditions, such as elevated cholesterol levels and hypertension. Intermittent fasting has demonstrated the ability to decrease levels of both cholesterol and blood pressure, even in the absence of significant weight reduction. If you have observed a gradual increase in your numerical values during annual medical check-ups, it is possible that you can effectively reduce them through fasting, without significant weight loss.

The concept of intermittent fasting may not be advisable for every woman. Individuals with a distinct health condition or a predisposition towards hypoglycemia should seek guidance from a medical professional. Notwithstanding, this emergent dietary phenomenon presents distinct advantages for females who inherently exhibit greater fat deposition in their bodies and may encounter difficulties in eliminating such fat reservoirs.

The Impact Of Intermittent Fasting On Weight Reduction

The human body accumulates and retains excess calories in the form of adipose tissue. When commencing intermittent fasting, your body will undertake various physiological changes aimed at enhancing accessibility to its stored energy reserves. Outlined below are a few modifications that occur within the human body. There has been a decrease in the production of insulin. Upon consumption of food, there is a noticeable increase in insulin levels. Thus, while fasting, there is a decline in the levels of insulin.

During the period of fasting, there is an increase in the concentration of human growth hormone (HGH) which facilitates fat reduction and promotes the development of lean muscle mass. The nervous system dispatches norepinephrine to adipocytes within the body, with the purpose of metabolizing fats into adipose-derived energy to facilitate the production of energy.

During the period of intermittent fasting, it will become evident that there is a decrease in the quantity of calories ingested. This primary factor elucidates how intermittent fasting effectively promotes weight reduction. Each of the various manifestations of intermittent fasting necessitates the omission of meals. Unless and unless there is an attempt to excessively increase food intake within the designated eating window, the result will be a reduction in overall calorie consumption.

Additionally, incorporating intermittent fasting into one's routine can contribute to the reduction of abdominal fat. Please ensure to conduct weekly self-assessments. The advantages of intermittent fasting extend beyond mere weight reduction. You need not be excessively concerned with calorie counting. Nevertheless, this does not imply that you have the permission to consume various types of unhealthy food. Partake of sustenance in the manner befitting your customary daily routine. Maintain a nutritious diet and ensure an ample intake of protein while avoiding detrimental carbohydrates and sugars.

One of the primary advantages inherent in this dietary approach is its inherent simplicity. As an example, let us contemplate the utilization of the 16/8 method. Within this particular approach, a designated time frame of 8 hours is allotted for consumption of food. Instead of partaking in the consumption of three or more meals in a given day, you will now engage in the consumption of only two meals. This not only facilitates a simpler lifestyle, but also enhances the ease of maintenance. It is advisable to select a dietary approach that you can maintain consistently over an extended period. If you ensure that you maintain a nutritious diet while adhering to the program, you will indeed be able to achieve weight loss. Minimize your consumption of carbohydrates and sugar to the greatest extent possible. Rather, opt for nutrient-rich sources of protein and foods that contain healthy fats. By allowing your body a respite between meals, it is afforded ample time to effectively metabolize the calories recently ingested.

LEAN MUSCLE GAIN

You may harbor inquiries concerning the intermittent protocol and its potential impact on your muscle mass. You will continue to experience muscle development while adhering to this dietary regimen. There are three factors that it is imperative for you to bear in mind. Continue reading to gain further insight.

The choice of intermittent fasting method appropriate for you is contingent upon the nature of your lifestyle. Based on your specific requirements, be it of a spiritual or physical nature, you have the option to choose a specific fasting approach. Irrespective of the motives behind commencing this dietary regimen, one may inquire about the methods by which muscle can be developed while adhering to the intermittent fasting protocols. There is a prevalent misconception that the development of muscle is unattainable, however, this notion couldn't be further from reality. There are several actions that one can undertake in order to optimize their chances of achieving success.

If you observe a specific fasting period, such as abstaining from food between 5 a.m. and 7 p.m., it would be advantageous to incorporate your exercise regimen into the evening timeframe. It would not be feasible to rise prior to 5 am. It is equally necessary to consume a meal prior to initiating resistance training, and it is not advisable to partake in exercise during the afternoon hours. After engaging in physical activity, it is imperative that you partake in the consumption of proteins and carbohydrates in order to initiate the process of recuperation. If one is engaged in evening training, it is possible to conveniently fit in a light meal post-workout. You have the option to engage in a physical exercise routine for a duration of one hour, subsequently allowing your body to recuperate before retiring to slumber.

It is advisable to structure your meals in a manner where the majority of the calories you are recommended to consume are immediately following your physical exercise session. It is vital that you undertake this action, as during this juncture your physique will effectively utilize these calories to foster the development of lean muscle mass and expedite the process of recovery. You are required to ascertain the precise caloric intake necessary for muscle development. It is essential to consume 20% of those calories before engaging in physical exercise. This should consist of a combination of proteins and carbohydrates. An additional 60% of the overall calorie intake should be ingested during the post-workout time frame. You have the option of dividing this into two smaller meals, should that be your preference, and distributing it across the subsequent couple of hours. Your calorie consumption will undoubtedly be elevated, and you have the opportunity to maximize your calorie intake by selecting foods that are particularly calorie-dense, such as oats and red meats, among other options. Ensure that you are ingesting nutrient-dense carbohydrates following your exercise session. This would furnish your body with the requisite caloric intake to initiate the process of recuperation. There is no need for you to be concerned about completely eliminating fats from your meals. Alternatively, you may opt to partake in a substantial meal containing a significant amount of carbohydrates or proteins directly following your training session, followed by a meal high in fats or proteins prior to retiring to bed. Nonetheless, it is imperative to ensure that your post-workout meal is comprised of a diminished amount of fat. Fatty substances contain a significant amount of energy, making it more feasible to consume them in larger quantities, such as nuts and oils. This is a more convenient alternative to consuming carbohydrates when experiencing a feeling of satiety.

Conclusively, it is imperative to bear in mind an additional factor when practicing intermittent fasting and aiming to cultivate muscular strength. Upon waking up, it is advisable to consume a meal. If you are engaging in fasting solely for reasons of convenience, it is advisable to consume a meal corresponding to your usual waking hour. It is advisable to partake in nourishment prior to commencing your fasting period. We recommend incorporating protein sources with a slower digestion rate into your diet, such as red meat and cottage cheese. This meal should represent 20% of your daily caloric consumption. Additionally, some carbohydrates and fats may be incorporated into this meal. This dietary intervention will supply your body with the essential amino acids required to sustain you during the fasting period. If you so desire, you may choose to return to a state of slumber. Nonetheless, the inconvenience of having to awaken for sustenance and subsequently return to slumber would present a burdensome ordeal. This is not a sustainable proposition in the long term. It is advisable to strategize your planning in a manner that allows your body to acclimate to this established eating schedule. If one were accustomed to arising early in the morning, this task would be rather effortless. There is no necessity for you to make any additional modifications to your schedule. This would be a suitable addition.

Ensure that these tips have been duly considered. Engaging in rigorous physical activity while adhering to a reduced calorie intake as a result of prolonged fasting is likely to yield unfavorable outcomes. You will ultimately exhaust yourself and subsequently deprive your body of the essential glucose needed to initiate the recuperative phase. After a certain period of time, the depletion of glycogen from your body would not yield favorable outcomes. In order to mitigate this issue, it will be necessary for you to adapt to consuming meals with more forcefulness. Over time, your body will acclimate to this sensation, gradually perceiving it as the new baseline. Therefore, exercise patience and allow yourself sufficient time to acclimate.

Chapter 6: Anticipated Outcomes During the Period of Fasting

Similar to any alteration in your daily regimen, you will need to make certain concessions throughout your period of fasting. During the initial phases of adjustment, one may experience certain periods of discomfort while acclimating to the unfamiliar eating regimen. Fortunately, the majority of fasts are of relatively brief duration. Except if you have specifically opted for an extended fasting approach, you have the freedom to incorporate fasting into your routine to any desired extent. Thus, during the periods of fasting, it is imperative to possess an understanding of how your body is expected to react.

You will continue to experience food cravings. Make an earnest effort to disregard their presence. In order to mitigate the impact of cravings, engage yourself in activities that occupy your mind and prevent excessive contemplation of food. Indeed, endeavor to schedule the days during which your food consumption will be minimal in alignment with those in which you will be occupied with numerous tasks, in consideration of this rationale. Avoid perceiving it as "depriving yourself" or engaging in starvation, as you are well aware that this approach is temporary and intended for long-lasting achievements. You will not experience a perpetual state of absence, and you can strategically schedule your fasting days to accommodate your social engagements, thus ensuring your presence at both Mike's birthday and Jess' farewell event.

Your eating pattern will be modified. While this may be self-evident, please remember to bear this in mind throughout the course of your workday. In the event that you are observing a full day of fasting and are unexpectedly confronted with a delectable meal during lunch, it will be necessary for you to exercise restraint, unless you are willing to modify your entire fasting schedule or postpone fasting altogether (as there is never an opportune moment to commence). Additionally, taking into account your schedule, which may be influenced by work commitments, parental responsibilities, sporting activities, and similar factors, it may be necessary for you to make adaptations in terms of meal timings. This encompasses lunch, as well as dinner in the company of your family or your post-workout meal. Anticipate experiencing occasional hunger or diminished overall appetite.

The latter is significant because adhering to proper refueling requires consuming meals at their designated times, regardless of current feelings of hunger or lack thereof. It is recommended that one interrupts their fasting cycle, as it is possible to develop a diminished appetite and eventually lose the inclination to eat. Although this may seem implausible at present, it does occur.

There will be a disparity in the timing of your return to your residence compared to previous occurrences. It is conceivable that you and your romantic partner would partake in watching films and indulging in refreshments at 10 o'clock in the evening on Fridays. Having commenced an intermittent fasting regimen, you have chosen to cease consumption of food by 8 pm daily. What to do? Talk to your partner. The individual in question will possess an understanding of your objectives. If you highly regard those M&Ms on Friday, then you might want to contemplate adopting an alternative day fasting approach to accommodate this indulgence. Another option to consider is altering your designated time frame for eating, so that it begins at a later hour to accommodate longer periods of wakefulness on weekends.

Additional scenarios that you might encounter include alterations in the designated meal schedules, unexpected indulgences, or uneasiness experienced from consuming specific food items subsequent to a period of abstinence. Your digestive system may undergo some changes in its processing of food following a period of fasting, thus leading to occasions when previously enjoyed indulgences no longer agree with your stomach or gastrointestinal system. With the passage of time, you will come to learn about this phenomenon (as not everyone may encounter it), so it is important to be prepared for the occurrence of unfamiliar bowel movements or cramps resulting from the consumption of food that is no longer part of your regular diet.

What types of physical activities can be performed during a period of fasting?

It is indeed possible and advisable to engage in exercise while fasting. What type of exercise performed while fasting would yield optimal results? A moderate response is the prevailing consensus. It is advisable to adhere to shorter duration workout sessions in order to prevent the loss of muscle mass, as opposed to fat. You certainly wouldn't want to relinquish the muscle you've diligently built. Fasting induces a physiological state wherein the optimization of calorie utilization during exercise becomes crucial. Therefore, akin to the majority of rigorous exercise regimens, wherein one expends all their stored energy to execute forceful lifts and achieve personal records, it is viable to consider incorporating branch chain amino acids (BCAA) as a supplementary measure during your workout session, aiming to counteract the inherent risk of muscle deterioration.

If one is engaging in rigorous exercise regimes, it is advisable to limit their duration. The temporal aspect is of utmost importance in this context. Participating in marathons will be beyond your capability. However, you can engage in shorter, yet intense weightlifting or cardiovascular sessions.

Furthermore, in order to optimize fuel efficiency and facilitate the burning of fat, it is advised to consume food immediately following your workout sessions. Indeed, you have correctly comprehended this information: it is advised that you consume a meal promptly after engaging in physical exercise. Consequently, you will be engaging in your exercise routine while in a state of fasting.

The advantages of engaging in physical activity during a period of fasting are as follows:

- Enhanced explosive performance (e.g., quick sprints, vertical jumps, etc.).
- Augmented explosive capabilities (e.g., rapid sprints, dynamic jumps, etc.).
- Amplified explosive output (e.g., burst sprints, explosive jumps, etc.).
- Heightened explosive reaction (e.g., rapid sprints, explosive leaps, etc.).
- Elevated explosive potential (e.g., swift sprints, powerful jumps, etc.).

- Enhanced vascular perfusion and circulation, coupled with your pre-existing optimized blood glucose and insulin reactivity, result in improved muscular engorgement and enhanced physiological adaptation to physical activity (however, it is important to note that this effect can also be achieved through alternative combinations of proper nutrition and exercise).

- Enhanced lipid metabolism and reduction in adipose tissue.

- Enhanced functioning of the endocrine system.
- Improved regulation and response of the endocrine system.
- Enhanced physiological response of the

endocrine system. • Enhanced endocrine system functionality. • Heightened endocrine system response.

• Enhance the development of lean muscle tissue.

• Enhanced physical composition.

Physical exercises serve as an enhancer for the physiological impacts that fasting can induce on the human body. When appropriately timed, such as during a fasted workout, you can expect to observe enhancements in the specific areas that you are already focusing on during your fasting period.

Ensure that your exercise sessions are approximately 45 minutes in duration in order to prevent excessive strain on your body. No one wants regression. Provided that you adhere to these guidelines, consume nourishing food upon concluding your fast, and adequately hydrate yourself, you can expect to achieve consistent outcomes in your workout sessions. There should be no decline in performance, nor should you experience any feelings of general weakness or fatigue during this time. If such is the case, you may need to consider one of two courses of action: increase your caloric intake (if you are practicing alternate day fasting, it may be advisable to limit yourself to only one 24-hour fast) or reduce the frequency or intensity of your workouts. Exercise self-monitoring and maintain regular communication with your healthcare providers (physicians, trainers, etc.) for guidance and support.

What Kind of Progress Should You See?

Similar to any new dietary or physical fitness regimen, it is anticipated that there may be variations in your progress over the course of the week. In general, it can be anticipated that an individual will experience a reduction in body weight ranging from 3-8%, along with a corresponding decrease in waist circumference, during the initial 3-12 weeks. Nevertheless, it is crucial to bear in mind that solely relying on intermittent fasting will not yield the desired outcomes. It is imperative to complement it with a suitable nutrition plan.

Moreover, it is important to keep in mind that there may be initial fluctuations. Nevertheless, as time progresses, it is anticipated that individuals will experience a reduction in weight, regardless of the approach they have employed. The process of weight loss ought to be gradual, and although certain fasting methods may lead to more significant weight loss (potentially resulting in muscle loss - if this is a concern, I recommend sticking with the 16:8 method), you should observe these effects regardless of the specific fasting plan you have selected.

Provided that you adhere to a suitable resistance training regimen, it is likely that you will observe a reduction in adipose tissue alongside a corresponding enhancement in muscular development as your body reaches equilibrium. Your attire may exhibit a distinct alteration, your physical movements may undergo a transformation, and your culinary preferences may even experience a shift as your gustatory senses undergo rejuvenation through the practice of fasting.

Following a period of approximately one week of fasting, it should become evident that one's hunger levels have diminished compared to previous levels. Your physiology has undergone adjustments in response to the revised eating schedule, enabling you to navigate through your fasts with relatively greater ease. Indeed, your body will have ceased desiring sustenance during its previous accustomed feeding periods and will now yearn for nourishment according to the new schedule imposed upon it. This demonstrates significant advancement as it indicates that your body is acclimating, thereby facilitating a smoother continuation of your fasting routine.

If your mood has not reached stability within approximately ten days, it is necessary to contemplate one of the aforementioned alternatives we have previously discussed: either modify your fasting regimen by reducing the number of fasting days or lower the intensity of your workout routine.

It is possible that you may need to alter the scheduling of your activities. It is possible that your level of focus may have diminished in the afternoon compared to earlier periods. I would suggest endeavoring to allocate those activities to the morning hours, when your cognitive capabilities are at their sharpest. You are likely to observe an improvement in lucidity as a result of streamlining your dietary regimen and implementing suitable modifications to counteract the adverse consequences associated with excessive fat accumulation in your body such as fatigue, difficulties in concentration, and so forth.

Advantages of practicing Intermittent Fasting

Given the various advantages of fasting, there exist individuals who are employing this practice to both achieve weight reduction and to address their health concerns. Additionally, certain individuals posit that fasting can be employed as a means to retain a youthful appearance and extend one's lifespan. Therefore, I find this procedure to be intriguing. The plain truth is that I would like to discuss the advantages of intermittent fasting with you for the same reasons.

Truly, this method of consumption is not particularly difficult. The act of being accused in a court setting can be likened to consuming all that is required for sustenance in a single day, only to abstain from any nourishment overnight. It signifies the absence of food, except for water. This stands in stark contrast to our customary dietary practices. Nevertheless, fasting can be perceived as a drastic method for achieving weight-loss. Nonetheless, it is an effective approach for individuals to achieve both physical and emotional well-being.

Intermittent fasting has the potential to enhance mental clarity and fortify both the physical and spiritual aspects of one's being. While it is widely held among the general populace that extended periods of food deprivation are detrimental to health, scientific research has unequivocally substantiated the numerous advantages of Intermittent Fasting.

It effectively eliminates the urge for food and sugar consumption.

Frequently, the sensation of "hunger" is often attributable to a yearning for sugars and carbohydrates. During periods of fasting, the body undergoes a metabolic shift whereby it transitions from relying on carbohydrates as a source of energy to utilizing stored fat reserves for fuel. Your body will acquire the knowledge that carbohydrates are unnecessary for energy and will utilize the stored fat within your body for energy production.

In addition to mitigating your desires for sugar, you will also eliminate your cravings for the specific sustenance. Since the body will recognize that it does not require food for energy, it will not frequently experience cravings for it. Therefore, by eliminating all sources of hunger, you will successfully navigate through the day. This is the reason why the notion of consuming meals 5-6 times a day is unfounded. By consuming meals at a frequency of 5-6 times per day and incorporating carbohydrates into your diet, you effectively hinder your body's ability to engage in the fat-burning process. This is attributed to the fact that the human body tends to prioritize the utilization of carbohydrates as its primary source of energy prior to turning to the stored fat reserves within the body.

It enhances insulin sensitivity

Insulin is an endogenous hormone that governs the cellular functionality within the human body. The pancreas produces insulin and releases it in response to food consumption. Subsequently, it attaches to signaling cells and facilitates the storage of sugars in our body as a source of energy. The reduction in insulin requirements for storing these sugars directly corresponds to an increase in our insulin sensitivity, thereby enabling more optimal and sustained functionality of insulin.

When we consume meals or snacks on a frequent basis, ranging from 5 to 6 times within a day, our insulin levels experience an extended duration of elevated presence. This insulin will not be optimally utilized, thereby leading to the gradual development of resistance towards it. The development of type 2 diabetes or prediabetes can occur when there is resistance to the effects of insulin. Diabetes is a medical condition characterized by impaired sugar storage due to inadequate functioning of pancreatic-produced insulin. In the event of this occurrence, the sugars will not undergo storage as a source of energy and instead will persist within our circulatory system, resulting in elevated levels of blood sugar and arterial calcification.

This can ultimately lead to the development of conditions such as kidney diseases, cardiac incidents, erectile dysfunction, visual impairments, strokes, nerve impairment, and an array of other serious health complications. Nevertheless, protracted periods of fasting necessitate the body to rely on its fat stores for energy rather than the ingested food being digested. This will facilitate a reduction in insulin production by your body, subsequently promoting enhanced insulin sensitivity, thereby mitigating the occurrence of these resultant issues.

Intermittent fasting is a straightforward practice.

It necessitates minimal exertion to strategically coordinate the portion, caliber, and schedule of your meals. Dedicated gym enthusiasts devote considerable effort to meticulously preparing their meals in order to monitor their caloric intake. This approach is deemed acceptable in isolation, but it has the potential to deplete considerable energy and consume a significant amount of time.

In the present era, as a result of our increasingly rapid and demanding patterns of living, time has become a scarce resource. Consequently, it is prudent to optimize time management by removing superfluous responsibilities such as meal preparation. During the period of fasting, one's primary concern rests upon selecting and organizing one or two meals, with the assurance of predetermined meal times throughout the day. This will enable you to allocate a greater proportion of your time to tasks of higher significance.

Upon recognizing that meal prepping holds relatively limited significance, one shall observe that comparable outcomes can be achieved with reduced exertion. This phenomenon is commonly referred to as the principle of 80/20. A significant majority (80%) of our outcomes are derived from a comparatively small proportion (20%) of our endeavors. It is incumbent upon us to determine the crucial 20%. Frequently, the act of food preparation in advance does not pertain to the minority 20%.

Additionally, as you consume one or two sizable meals per day, there is no need to consistently monitor your calorie intake. Furthermore, it presents a notably arduous task to surpass your recommended daily calorie intake within a limited span of one or two meals, unless, of course, your food choices consist primarily of unhealthy options.

Please be advised that the information provided is not applicable to individuals who are considered professional bodybuilders. One cannot anticipate achieving success in competitions without maintaining optimal levels of leanness. Therefore, I strongly advise individuals who are participating in competitions to meticulously monitor their calorie intake and steadfastly adhere to proven strategies."

It exhibits adaptability

Maintaining stringent dietary plans can pose considerable challenges in terms of long-term viability. The majority of us are engaged in significant and arduous occupations that restrict our ability to consume meals as necessary. Instead, we are granted intervals at times that are not necessarily essential. Alternatively, our frequent travels often prevent us from consuming our meals at the appropriate times. Nevertheless, fasting offers a significant degree of flexibility. Due to the limited temporal availability, you are afforded the liberty to select the timing of your meals. This will provide you with the chance to consume meals at your utmost convenience.

Personally, I find it exceedingly challenging to effectively plan my meals and adhere to my designated meal schedule whilst in transit or fulfilling professional obligations. Fasting enables me to abstain from consuming food for extended periods, and selectively eat at my preferred convenience.

Benefits to One's Well-being

Research indicates that Intermittent Fasting has a multitude of positive effects on health. Individuals who are overweight or suffer from diseases like diabetes may benefit the most from Intermittent Fasting.

Individuals who are overweight or have been diagnosed with type 2 diabetes will experience greater weight loss and enhanced cardiovascular well-being through periodic fasting. Even if they opt to maintain their current calorie intake instead of reducing it, they will still observe noticeable outcomes. Certainly, if you desire to optimize your outcomes, it is imperative to maintain a slight caloric deficit while consuming nutritious dietary choices.

Additional health advantages include: Another health benefit to consider is: Furthermore, there are other positive implications for health, such as: Moreover, there are additional reasons to prioritize health, including: In addition to these, there are other notable health benefits, such as: Additionally, it is important to acknowledge the various health advantages, such as:

- Restricting the occurrence of inflammation
- Lowering blood pressure
- Enhance pancreatic function • Optimize pancreatic function • Boost pancreatic function • Increase pancreatic function • Refined pancreatic function • Enhance the functioning of the pancreas
- Provides defense against the onset of cardiovascular disease
- Decrease overall cholesterol and LDL concentrations
- Enhances insulin sensitivity • Enhances the body's response to insulin • Increases insulin sensitivity • Augments insulin sensitivity • Boosts insulin sensitivity • Elevates insulin sensitivity

Although Intermittent Fasting is generally considered beneficial for individuals with diabetes, it can potentially have adverse effects as it involves restricting nutrient intake during specific periods of the day. Once again, it is advisable to consult with your physician prior to implementing Intermittent Fasting as a healthy practice for individuals with diabetes.

Accelerated Bodily Mass Reduction

As previously mentioned, typically the energy derived from the carbohydrates consumed is what sustains the body. This will inhibit the utilization of the adipose reserves within your body. However, during the state of fasting, one exercises the body's ability to utilize its stored fat as a source of energy. This, in isolation, will result in immediate and expeditious reduction in body fat, thereby enhancing both aesthetic appearance and overall well-being.

Furthermore, the act of fasting for one to two days per week inherently leads to a substantial reduction in calorie intake, amounting to an estimated range of 1000 to 4500 calories on a weekly basis.

This will lead to significant and swift reduction in weight, enabling you to lose an approximate range of 0.5-1 pound per week. Moreover, you will effectively retain your muscle mass while shedding fat, thereby facilitating remarkable physical enhancements.

Enhances Cognitive Function

Intermittent fasting also offers numerous advantages for cognitive function. It enhances memory functionality and expedites the process of acquiring knowledge. Additionally, it increases the production of Brain Derived Neurotropic Factor (BDNF), leading to the growth and development of brain tissues. This will enhance your cognitive capabilities and facilitate the development of robust musculature.

"Several additional advantages include:

Mitigates the Onset of Depression

Studies have demonstrated a correlation between decreased levels of brain-derived neurotrophic factor (BDNF) and the manifestation of depressive symptoms. A comprehensive investigation was undertaken using two mice afflicted with Alzheimer's disease in order to study the positive effects on cognitive function. One of the mice adhered to a regimen known as Intermittent Fasting, while the other mouse maintained a standard diet with an identical caloric intake.

They were subjected to the Morris water maze experiment, and the mouse that was practicing Intermittent Fasting navigated its way considerably more swiftly compared to the others.

Enhances the Generation of Ketones

Intermittent Fasting induces the active promotion of ketone synthesis. Ketones are acidic compounds synthesized by the human body to facilitate the utilization of fats as an energy substrate rather than relying on carbohydrates for energy production.

Efficient in mitigating brain trauma.

Fasting mitigates the adverse effects stemming from brain traumas, encompassing mitochondrial dysfunction, oxidative stress, and cognitive decline.

Mitigates the occurrence of Huntington's Disease

This condition will cause a reduction in your brain-derived neurotrophic factor (BDNF) levels, however, studies have demonstrated that rats with Huntington's disease maintained stable BDNF levels when subjected to periods of fasting.

www.ingramcontent.com/pod-product-compliance
Lightning Source LLC
Chambersburg PA
CBHW070031040426
42333CB00040B/1427